LOW OXALATE RECIPE BOOK

Kidney-Friendly Meals for a Healthy Lifestyle

Dr Lily Morgan

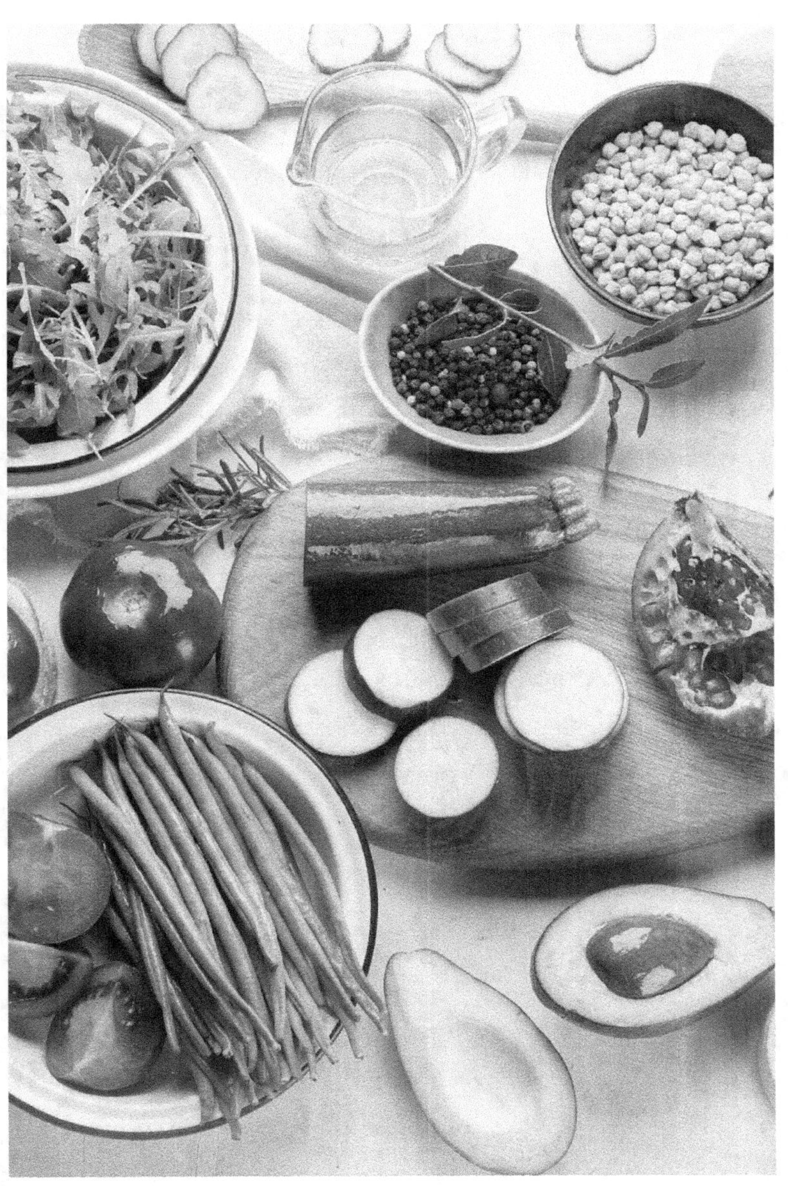

TABLE OF CONTENTS

Chapter 3: Lunch Recipes 37

Chapter 4: Dinner Recipes 53

Chapter 5: Snacks and Appetizers 69

Chapter 6: Desserts 81

INTRODUCTION

Oxalates, naturally occurring compounds found in various foods, are a topic often overlooked but of significant importance when it comes to our dietary choices. Understanding oxalates and their impact on our health is key to making informed decisions about what we eat.

Oxalates are tiny crystals that can form in the body when they bind to minerals like calcium. While some oxalates are produced within our own bodies, a major source of dietary oxalates comes from the foods we consume. These compounds are prevalent in many otherwise healthy foods, including leafy greens like spinach and Swiss chard, as well as in nuts, beets, and even chocolate. They can also be found in certain grains, like quinoa.

So, what's the concern with oxalates? When oxalate crystals accumulate, they can lead to various health issues, the most common being kidney stones. These tiny crystals can bind together and create stones that may cause intense pain and discomfort when they pass through the urinary tract.

This brings us to the importance of a low oxalate diet. For individuals prone to kidney stones or those with specific medical conditions like hyperoxaluria, reducing oxalate intake can be crucial. A low oxalate diet aims to minimize the consumption of high-oxalate foods to prevent the formation of these troublesome crystals.

However, it's essential to strike a balance. Not all foods containing oxalates need to be eliminated from your diet entirely, as many of them also provide essential nutrients. Instead, a well-balanced approach involves moderating high-oxalate foods, increasing fluid intake, and ensuring an adequate intake of calcium, which can help bind to oxalates and reduce their absorption in the body.

In summary, understanding oxalates and their impact on health is a valuable step toward making informed dietary choices. While a low oxalate diet may be necessary for some individuals, it's essential to consult with a healthcare professional or registered dietitian to create a personalized plan that maintains a balance between health and enjoyment of food. By doing so, we can navigate the world of oxalates with knowledge and confidence.

Chapter 1: 30 Day Meal Plan

Week 1

Day 1:

- Breakfast: Low Oxalate Oatmeal
- Lunch: Chicken and Vegetable Stir-Fry
- Dinner: Baked Salmon with Lemon-Dill Sauce
- Snacks: Guacamole with Veggie Sticks
- Dessert: Low Oxalate Chocolate Brownies

Day 2:

- Breakfast: Spinach and Feta Breakfast Casserole
- Lunch: Quinoa Salad with Roasted Vegetables
- Dinner: Grilled Chicken with Pesto
- Snacks: Roasted Red Pepper and Feta Dip
- Dessert: Berry Parfait

Day 3:

- Breakfast: Blueberry Almond Pancakes
- Lunch: Tuna Salad Lettuce Wraps
- Dinner: Beef and Broccoli Stir-Fry

- Snacks: Deviled Eggs
- Dessert: Lemon Sorbet

Day 4:

- Breakfast: Scrambled Eggs with Herbs
- Lunch: Turkey and Avocado Wrap
- Dinner: Spaghetti Squash with Tomato Sauce
- Snacks: Cucumber Slices with Cream Cheese
- Dessert: Vanilla Chia Seed Pudding

Day 5:

- Breakfast: Avocado Toast with Tomato
- Lunch: Spinach and Strawberry Salad
- Dinner: Lemon Garlic Shrimp Scampi
- Snacks: Kale Chips
- Dessert: Almond Flour Sugar Cookies

Day 6:

- Breakfast: Greek Yogurt Parfait
- Lunch: Broccoli and Cheddar Soup
- Dinner: Stuffed Bell Peppers with Ground Turkey
- Snacks: Edamame with Sea Salt

- Dessert: Poached Pears in Red Wine

Day 7:

- Breakfast: Breakfast Burrito with Low Oxalate Veggies
- Lunch: Greek Salad with Grilled Chicken
- Dinner: Portobello Mushroom Steaks
- Snacks: Trail Mix with Low Oxalate Nuts
- Dessert: Chocolate Avocado Mousse

Week 2

Day 8:

- Breakfast: Banana Walnut Muffins
- Lunch: Cauliflower Fried Rice
- Dinner: Baked Cod with Herbed Crust
- Snacks: Carrot and Hummus
- Dessert: Baked Apples with Cinnamon

Day 9:

- Breakfast: Quinoa Breakfast Bowl
- Lunch: Lentil and Vegetable Soup
- Dinner: Zucchini Noodles with Pesto

- Snacks: Stuffed Mushrooms
- Dessert: Coconut Macaroons

Day 10:

- Breakfast: Berry Smoothie Bowl
- Lunch: Caprese Salad
- Dinner: Quinoa-Stuffed Acorn Squash
- Snacks: Greek Yogurt Dip with Veggies
- Dessert: Strawberry Shortcake

Day 11:

- Breakfast: Chia Seed Pudding
- Lunch: Shrimp and Asparagus Salad
- Dinner: Thai Green Curry with Tofu
- Snacks: Baked Sweet Potato Fries
- Dessert: Pumpkin Pie Bites

Day 12:

- Breakfast: Sweet Potato Hash
- Lunch: Roasted Red Pepper Hummus Wrap
- Dinner: Roasted Cauliflower Steak
- Snacks: Spinach and Artichoke Dip

- Dessert: Blueberry Almond Crisp

Day 13:

- Breakfast: Veggie Omelette
- Lunch: Spinach and Mushroom Quesadilla
- Dinner: Turkey Meatballs in Tomato Sauce
- Snacks: Almond and Coconut Energy Bites
- Dessert: Banana Ice Cream

Day 14:

- Breakfast: Coconut Milk Rice Pudding
- Lunch: Cucumber and Dill Salad
- Dinner: Sweet Potato and Black Bean Chili
- Snacks: Mini Caprese Skewers
- Dessert: Lemon Poppy Seed Cake

Week 3

Day 15:

- Breakfast: Cottage Cheese Pancakes
- Lunch: Turkey and Spinach Stuffed Bell Peppers
- Dinner: Lemon Herb Tilapia
- Snacks: Crispy Chickpeas

- Dessert: Rice Pudding with Berries

Day 16:

- Breakfast: Zucchini Bread
- Lunch: Eggplant and Tomato Stack
- Dinner: Ratatouille
- Snacks: Avocado Deviled Eggs
- Dessert: Dark Chocolate Bark with Nuts

Day 17:

- Breakfast: Almond Butter Toast
- Lunch: Chickpea and Cucumber Salad
- Dinner: BBQ Pulled Chicken Lettuce Wraps
- Snacks: Smoked Salmon Roll-Ups
- Dessert: Mango Sorbet

Day 18:

- Breakfast: Green Smoothie
- Lunch: Creamy Butternut Squash Soup
- Dinner: Cabbage Roll Casserole
- Snacks: Pita Chips with Roasted Red Pepper Hummus

- Dessert: Pecan Pie Bites

Day 19:

- Breakfast: Low Oxalate Oatmeal
- Lunch: Chicken and Vegetable Stir-Fry
- Dinner: Baked Salmon with Lemon-Dill Sauce
- Snacks: Guacamole with Veggie Sticks
- Dessert: Low Oxalate Chocolate Brownies

Day 20:

- Breakfast: Spinach and Feta Breakfast Casserole
- Lunch: Quinoa Salad with Roasted Vegetables
- Dinner: Grilled Chicken with Pesto
- Snacks: Roasted Red Pepper and Feta Dip
- Dessert: Berry Parfait

Day 21:

- Breakfast: Blueberry Almond Pancakes
- Lunch: Tuna Salad Lettuce Wraps
- Dinner: Beef and Broccoli Stir-Fry
- Snacks: Deviled Eggs
- Dessert: Lemon Sorbet

Week 4

Day 22:

- Breakfast: Scrambled Eggs with Herbs
- Lunch: Turkey and Avocado Wrap
- Dinner: Spaghetti Squash with Tomato Sauce
- Snacks: Cucumber Slices with Cream Cheese
- Dessert: Vanilla Chia Seed Pudding

Day 23:

- Breakfast: Avocado Toast with Tomato
- Lunch: Spinach and Strawberry Salad
- Dinner: Lemon Garlic Shrimp Scampi
- Snacks: Kale Chips
- Dessert: Almond Flour Sugar Cookies

Day 24:

- Breakfast: Greek Yogurt Parfait
- Lunch: Broccoli and Cheddar Soup
- Dinner: Stuffed Bell Peppers with Ground Turkey
- Snacks: Edamame with Sea Salt
- Dessert: Poached Pears in Red Wine

Day 25:

- Breakfast: Breakfast Burrito with Low Oxalate Veggies
- Lunch: Greek Salad with Grilled Chicken
- Dinner: Portobello Mushroom Steaks
- Snacks: Trail Mix with Low Oxalate Nuts
- Dessert: Chocolate Avocado Mousse

Day 26:

- Breakfast: Banana Walnut Muffins
- Lunch: Cauliflower Fried Rice
- Dinner: Baked Cod with Herbed Crust
- Snacks: Carrot and Hummus
- Dessert: Baked Apples with Cinnamon

Day 27:

- Breakfast: Quinoa Breakfast Bowl
- Lunch: Lentil and Vegetable Soup
- Dinner: Zucchini Noodles with Pesto
- Snacks: Stuffed Mushrooms
- Dessert: Coconut Macaroons

Day 28:

- Breakfast: Berry Smoothie Bowl
- Lunch: Caprese Salad
- Dinner: Quinoa-Stuffed Acorn Squash
- Snacks: Greek Yogurt Dip with Veggies
- Dessert: Strawberry Shortcake

Day 29:

- Breakfast: Chia Seed Pudding
- Lunch: Shrimp and Asparagus Salad
- Dinner: Thai Green Curry with Tofu
- Snacks: Baked Sweet Potato Fries
- Dessert: Pumpkin Pie Bites

Day 30:

- Breakfast: Sweet Potato Hash
- Lunch: Roasted Red Pepper Hummus Wrap
- Dinner: Roasted Cauliflower Steak
- Snacks: Spinach and Artichoke Dip
- Dessert: Blueberry Almond Crisp

This completes the 30-day meal plan with a variety of low oxalate recipes for each day. Enjoy your journey to healthier eating!

Chapter 2: Breakfast Recipes

In Chapter 2 of our Low Oxalate Recipe Book, we're diving into the most important meal of the day – breakfast! These nutritious and delicious breakfast recipes are thoughtfully crafted to fit within a low oxalate diet while ensuring your mornings start with a burst of flavor and energy.

Low Oxalate Oatmeal

Ingredients:

- 1/2 cup rolled oats
- 1 cup almond milk
- 1 tablespoon honey
- 1/4 cup sliced strawberries
- 1 tablespoon chopped almonds

Instructions:

1. In a saucepan, combine rolled oats and almond milk.
2. Cook over medium heat until oats are tender, stirring occasionally.

3. Drizzle with honey and top with strawberries and chopped almonds.

Spinach and Feta Breakfast Casserole

Ingredients:

- 6 eggs
- 1 cup fresh spinach, chopped
- 1/2 cup crumbled feta cheese
- 1/4 cup diced red bell pepper
- Salt and pepper to taste

Instructions:

1. Preheat oven to 350°F (175°C).
2. In a bowl, beat the eggs and add spinach, feta, red bell pepper, salt, and pepper.
3. Pour the mixture into a greased baking dish and bake for 25-30 minutes or until set.

Blueberry Almond Pancakes

Ingredients:

- 1 cup almond flour
- 2 eggs
- 1/2 cup blueberries
- 1/4 teaspoon baking powder
- 1 tablespoon almond butter

Instructions:

1. In a bowl, mix almond flour, eggs, and baking powder.
2. Gently fold in blueberries.
3. Heat a non-stick skillet and spoon the batter onto it to make pancakes.
4. Serve with a dollop of almond butter.

Scrambled Eggs with Herbs

Ingredients:

- 4 eggs
- 2 tablespoons chopped fresh herbs (e.g., chives, parsley)

- Salt and pepper to taste

Instructions:

1. Crack eggs into a bowl and whisk.
2. Heat a skillet over medium heat, add eggs, herbs, salt, and pepper.
3. Cook, stirring gently until eggs are set but still moist.

Avocado Toast with Tomato

Ingredients:

- 2 slices of low oxalate bread
- 1 ripe avocado
- 1 tomato, sliced
- Salt and pepper to taste

Instructions:

1. Toast the bread slices.
2. Mash avocado and spread it on the toast.
3. Top with tomato slices, salt, and pepper.

Greek Yogurt Parfait

Ingredients:

- 1 cup Greek yogurt
- 1/4 cup low oxalate granola
- 1/2 cup mixed berries (e.g., strawberries, blueberries)

Instructions:

1. In a glass or bowl, layer Greek yogurt, granola, and mixed berries.
2. Repeat the layers until you reach the top.
3. Enjoy this delightful and nutritious parfait.

Breakfast Burrito with Low Oxalate Veggies

Ingredients:

- 2 large eggs
- 1/4 cup diced bell peppers
- 1/4 cup diced zucchini
- 2 tablespoons diced onion
- 2 tablespoons shredded cheddar cheese

- 1 whole-grain tortilla

Instructions:

1. In a skillet, sauté bell peppers, zucchini, and onion until tender.
2. Scramble the eggs in the same skillet.
3. Place the scrambled eggs and sautéed veggies on the tortilla, sprinkle with cheese, and roll it up.

Banana Walnut Muffins

Ingredients:

- 2 ripe bananas, mashed
- 2 eggs
- 1/4 cup walnut pieces
- 1 cup almond flour
- 1/4 cup honey
- 1/2 teaspoon baking soda

Instructions:

1. Preheat your oven to 350°F (175°C) and line a muffin tin with paper liners.

2. In a bowl, combine mashed bananas, eggs, honey, and almond flour. Mix until smooth.

3. Stir in walnut pieces and baking soda.

4. Fill each muffin cup 2/3 full with the batter and bake for 20-25 minutes until a toothpick comes out clean.

Quinoa Breakfast Bowl

Ingredients:

- 1 cup cooked quinoa
- 1/2 cup low-fat milk
- 1/4 cup fresh berries
- 1 tablespoon honey
- 1 tablespoon sliced almonds

Instructions:

1. Warm the cooked quinoa with milk in a saucepan over low heat.

2. Transfer to a bowl, top with fresh berries, drizzle with honey, and sprinkle with sliced almonds.

Berry Smoothie Bowl

Ingredients:

- 1 cup frozen mixed berries
- 1/2 cup Greek yogurt
- 1/4 cup low oxalate granola
- 1 tablespoon honey

Instructions:

1. Blend frozen berries and Greek yogurt until smooth.
2. Pour the smoothie into a bowl, top with granola, and drizzle with honey.

Chia Seed Pudding

Ingredients:

- 2 tablespoons chia seeds
- 1/2 cup almond milk
- 1/2 teaspoon vanilla extract
- 1 tablespoon maple syrup
- Fresh fruit for topping

Instructions:

1. Mix chia seeds, almond milk, vanilla extract, and maple syrup in a jar or bowl.

2. Refrigerate for a few hours or overnight until it thickens.

3. Top with fresh fruit before serving.

Sweet Potato Hash

Ingredients:

-   2 cups diced sweet potatoes

-   1/2 cup diced bell peppers

-   1/4 cup diced onions

-   2 tablespoons olive oil

-   Salt and pepper to taste

-   2 eggs (optional)

Instructions:

1. Heat olive oil in a skillet over medium-high heat.

2. Add sweet potatoes, bell peppers, and onions.

3. Sauté until sweet potatoes are tender and slightly crispy.

4. If desired, fry eggs separately and serve on top of the
    hash.

Veggie Omelette

Ingredients:

- 3 eggs
- 1/4 cup diced low oxalate veggies (e.g., spinach, mushrooms)
- 1/4 cup shredded cheese (choose low oxalate variety)
- Salt and pepper to taste

Instructions:

1. Whisk eggs in a bowl and season with salt and pepper.
2. Pour the egg mixture into a preheated, greased skillet.
3. Sprinkle diced veggies and cheese evenly over one half of the omelette.
4. Fold the other half over the fillings and cook until set.

Coconut Milk Rice Pudding

Ingredients:

- 1 cup cooked white rice
- 1 cup coconut milk
- 1/4 cup honey
- 1/4 teaspoon vanilla extract
- 1/4 teaspoon ground cinnamon

Instructions:

1. In a saucepan, combine cooked rice, coconut milk, honey, vanilla extract, and cinnamon.
2. Simmer on low heat, stirring occasionally, until the mixture thickens.
3. Serve warm or chilled.

Cottage Cheese Pancakes

Ingredients:

- 1 cup cottage cheese
- 2 eggs
- 1/4 cup almond flour
- 1 tablespoon honey

- 1/2 teaspoon vanilla extract

Instructions:

1. In a blender, combine cottage cheese, eggs, almond flour, honey, and vanilla extract.
2. Blend until smooth.
3. Cook pancake-sized portions on a griddle until golden brown on both sides.

Zucchini Bread

Ingredients:

- 2 cups grated zucchini
- 2 eggs
- 1/4 cup coconut oil
- 1/2 cup almond flour
- 1/2 cup coconut flour
- 1/4 cup honey
- 1 teaspoon cinnamon
- 1/2 teaspoon baking soda

Chapter 3: Lunch Recipes

Lunchtime can be a delightful part of your day, especially when you have a variety of low oxalate options at your fingertips. In this chapter, we'll explore a selection of lunch recipes that are not only nutritious but bursting with flavors.

Chicken and Vegetable Stir-Fry

Ingredients:

- 1 boneless, skinless chicken breast, thinly sliced
- 2 cups mixed vegetables (bell peppers, broccoli, snap peas)
- 2 tablespoons low-sodium soy sauce
- 1 tablespoon olive oil
- 1 teaspoon minced garlic
- 1/2 teaspoon ginger paste
- Salt and pepper to taste

Instructions:

1. Heat olive oil in a skillet over medium-high heat.
2. Add chicken slices and cook until no longer pink.

3. Stir in garlic and ginger, then add vegetables.

4. Drizzle with soy sauce and sauté until veggies are tender.

5. Season with salt and pepper and serve hot.

Quinoa Salad with Roasted Vegetables

Ingredients:

- 1 cup quinoa, cooked and cooled
- 2 cups mixed roasted vegetables (zucchini, bell peppers, carrots)
- 1/4 cup chopped fresh herbs (parsley, basil)
- 2 tablespoons olive oil
- 2 tablespoons lemon juice
- Salt and pepper to taste

Instructions:

1. In a large bowl, combine quinoa and roasted vegetables.

2. In a separate bowl, whisk together olive oil, lemon juice, herbs, salt, and pepper.

3. Pour the dressing over the quinoa and veggies, toss well, and chill before serving.

Tuna Salad Lettuce Wraps

Ingredients:

- 1 can of low-sodium tuna, drained
- 2 tablespoons Greek yogurt
- 1 tablespoon Dijon mustard
- 1/4 cup diced celery
- 1/4 cup diced red onion
- Lettuce leaves for wrapping
- Salt and pepper to taste

Instructions:

1. In a bowl, mix tuna, Greek yogurt, mustard, celery, and red onion.
2. Season with salt and pepper.
3. Spoon the tuna salad onto lettuce leaves and enjoy your healthy wraps.

Turkey and Avocado Wrap

Ingredients:

- 4 large lettuce leaves
- 8 slices of turkey breast
- 1 avocado, sliced
- 1/4 cup shredded carrot
- 1/4 cup cucumber strips
- Hummus for spreading

Instructions:

1. Lay out the lettuce leaves and place turkey slices on each.
2. Add avocado slices, shredded carrot, and cucumber strips.
3. Spread hummus over the ingredients, then roll up the wraps.

Spinach and Strawberry Salad

Ingredients:

- 2 cups fresh spinach leaves
- 1 cup sliced strawberries

- 1/4 cup sliced almonds
- 2 tablespoons balsamic vinaigrette dressing
- Crumbled feta cheese (optional)

Instructions:

1. In a bowl, combine spinach, strawberries, and sliced almonds.
2. Drizzle with balsamic vinaigrette dressing and top with crumbled feta if desired.

Broccoli and Cheddar Soup

Ingredients:

- 2 cups chopped broccoli florets
- 1 cup shredded low oxalate cheddar cheese
- 1 small onion, diced
- 2 cups low-sodium vegetable broth
- 1 cup almond milk
- 2 tablespoons olive oil
- Salt and pepper to taste

Instructions:

1. In a pot, sauté diced onion in olive oil until translucent.
2. Add broccoli, vegetable broth, and almond milk. Simmer until broccoli is tender.
3. Use an immersion blender to blend the soup until smooth.
4. Stir in shredded cheddar cheese until melted.
5. Season with salt and pepper and serve hot.

Greek Salad with Grilled Chicken

Ingredients:

- 2 boneless, skinless chicken breasts, grilled and sliced
- 2 cups mixed greens
- 1 cup cherry tomatoes, halved
- 1/2 cucumber, sliced
- 1/4 cup Kalamata olives
- 1/4 cup crumbled low oxalate feta cheese
- Greek dressing (olive oil, lemon juice, oregano)

Instructions:

1. Arrange mixed greens on a plate.

2. Top with grilled chicken, cherry tomatoes, cucumber, olives, and feta cheese.

3. Drizzle with Greek dressing and enjoy this Mediterranean delight.

Cauliflower Fried Rice

Ingredients:

- 2 cups cauliflower rice
- 1/2 cup diced bell peppers
- 1/2 cup diced carrots
- 1/2 cup peas
- 2 tablespoons low-sodium soy sauce
- 1 tablespoon sesame oil
- 2 eggs, beaten (optional)
- Green onions for garnish

Instructions:

1. In a pan, sauté bell peppers, carrots, and peas in sesame oil.

2. Add cauliflower rice and cook until tender.

3. Push the rice to one side, scramble eggs on the other side (if using).

4. Stir in soy sauce, mix well, and garnish with green onions.

Lentil and Vegetable Soup

Ingredients:

- 1 cup green or brown lentils, rinsed
- 4 cups low-sodium vegetable broth
- 1 cup diced tomatoes
- 1 cup diced celery
- 1 cup diced carrots
- 1 cup diced onion
- 2 cloves garlic, minced
- 1 teaspoon dried thyme
- Salt and pepper to taste

Instructions:

1. In a large pot, sauté onions, carrots, celery, and garlic until softened.

2. Add lentils, vegetable broth, tomatoes, and thyme.

3. Simmer for 20-25 minutes until lentils are tender.

4. Season with salt and pepper and serve hot.

Caprese Salad

Ingredients:

- 2 large ripe tomatoes, sliced
- 1 cup fresh low oxalate mozzarella, sliced
- Fresh basil leaves
- Extra-virgin olive oil
- Balsamic glaze
- Salt and pepper to taste

Instructions:

1. Arrange tomato and mozzarella slices on a plate, alternating.
2. Tuck fresh basil leaves between the slices.
3. Drizzle with olive oil and balsamic glaze.
4. Season with salt and pepper for a simple, elegant salad.

Shrimp and Asparagus Salad

Ingredients:

- 1 cup cooked and peeled shrimp
- 1 cup cooked asparagus, chopped
- 1/2 cup cherry tomatoes, halved
- 1/4 cup sliced red onion
- 2 tablespoons lemon vinaigrette dressing
- Fresh parsley for garnish
- Salt and pepper to taste

Instructions:

1. Combine shrimp, asparagus, cherry tomatoes, and red onion in a bowl.
2. Drizzle with lemon vinaigrette dressing.
3. Season with salt and pepper, garnish with fresh parsley, and enjoy this light and refreshing salad.

Roasted Red Pepper Hummus Wrap

Ingredients:

- 1 whole-grain wrap
- 1/2 cup low oxalate roasted red pepper hummus

- 1 cup mixed greens
- 1/2 cup cucumber slices
- 1/4 cup shredded carrot
- 1/4 cup sliced black olives

Instructions:

1. Spread roasted red pepper hummus over the whole-grain wrap.
2. Layer on mixed greens, cucumber slices, shredded carrot, and black olives.
3. Roll up the wrap, slice in half, and savor the flavors.

Spinach and Mushroom Quesadilla

Ingredients:

- 2 whole-grain tortillas
- 1 cup fresh spinach leaves
- 1 cup sliced mushrooms
- 1/2 cup shredded low oxalate mozzarella cheese
- Olive oil for cooking

Instructions:

1. In a pan, sauté sliced mushrooms in olive oil until tender.
2. Place one tortilla in the pan, add spinach, mushrooms, and mozzarella cheese.
3. Top with the second tortilla and cook until cheese is melted and tortilla is crisp.
4. Slice into wedges and enjoy your quesadilla.

Cucumber and Dill Salad

Ingredients:

- 2 cucumbers, thinly sliced
- 1/4 cup Greek yogurt
- 1 tablespoon fresh dill, chopped
- 1 tablespoon lemon juice
- Salt and pepper to taste

Instructions:

1. In a bowl, combine cucumber slices, Greek yogurt, dill, and lemon juice.
2. Season with salt and pepper.
3. Chill before serving this refreshing cucumber salad.

Turkey and Spinach Stuffed Bell Peppers

Ingredients:

- 4 bell peppers, halved and seeded
- 1 pound ground turkey
- 2 cups fresh spinach, chopped
- 1 cup cooked quinoa
- 1/2 cup diced tomatoes
- 1/2 cup low oxalate tomato sauce
- 1/2 cup shredded low oxalate mozzarella cheese
- Italian seasoning, salt, and pepper

Instructions:

1. Preheat the oven to 375°F (190°C).
2. In a skillet, brown ground turkey and season with Italian seasoning, salt, and pepper.
3. Stir in spinach, cooked quinoa, diced tomatoes, and tomato sauce.
4. Fill each bell pepper half with the turkey mixture.
5. Top with shredded mozzarella cheese and bake for 25-30 minutes until peppers are tender and cheese is bubbly.

Eggplant and Tomato Stack

Ingredients:

- 1 large eggplant, sliced
- 2 large tomatoes, sliced
- 1/4 cup low oxalate goat cheese
- Fresh basil leaves
- Balsamic glaze
- Olive oil
- Salt and pepper to taste

Instructions:

1. Preheat your grill or grill pan.
2. Brush eggplant slices with olive oil and season with salt and pepper.
3. Grill eggplant and tomato slices until tender.
4. Assemble stacks with eggplant, tomato, and goat cheese.
5. Top with fresh basil leaves and drizzle with balsamic glaze.

Chickpea and Cucumber Salad

Ingredients:

- 2 cups canned chickpeas, rinsed and drained
- 1 cucumber, diced
- 1/4 cup red onion, finely chopped
- 1/4 cup fresh parsley, chopped
- 2 tablespoons olive oil
- 1 tablespoon lemon juice
- Salt and pepper to taste

Instructions:

1. In a bowl, combine chickpeas, cucumber, red onion, and fresh parsley.
2. Drizzle with olive oil and lemon juice.
3. Season with salt and pepper, toss gently, and serve this nutritious salad.

Creamy Butternut Squash Soup

Ingredients:

- 2 cups roasted butternut squash, mashed
- 1 cup low-sodium vegetable broth

- 1/2 cup unsweetened almond milk
- 1/2 teaspoon ground nutmeg
- Salt and pepper to taste

Instructions:

1. In a blender, combine mashed butternut squash, vegetable broth, almond milk, nutmeg, salt, and pepper.
2. Blend until smooth.
3. Transfer the mixture to a pot and heat until warmed through.
4. Serve this creamy soup with a sprinkle of nutmeg on top.

Chapter 4: Dinner Recipes

In this chapter, we delve into a delightful array of dinner recipes that are not only delicious but also low in oxalates. These recipes offer a variety of flavors and ingredients, ensuring that you'll never get bored with your low oxalate diet.

Baked Salmon with Lemon-Dill Sauce

Ingredients:

- 4 salmon fillets
- 2 tablespoons olive oil
- 1 lemon, juiced and zested
- 2 cloves garlic, minced
- 1 tablespoon fresh dill, chopped
- Salt and pepper to taste

Instructions:

1. Preheat your oven to 375°F (190°C).
2. Place salmon fillets on a baking sheet.

3. In a bowl, whisk together olive oil, lemon juice, lemon zest, garlic, dill, salt, and pepper.

4. Drizzle the lemon-dill sauce over the salmon.

5. Bake for 15-20 minutes until the salmon flakes easily with a fork.

Grilled Chicken with Pesto

Ingredients:

- 4 boneless, skinless chicken breasts
- 1/2 cup pesto sauce
- Salt and pepper to taste

Instructions:

1. Preheat your grill to medium-high heat.

2. Season chicken breasts with salt and pepper.

3. Grill the chicken for about 6-8 minutes per side until cooked through.

4. Brush pesto sauce over the chicken during the last few minutes of grilling.

Beef and Broccoli Stir-Fry

Ingredients:

- 1 pound lean beef, thinly sliced
- 2 cups broccoli florets
- 1/4 cup low-sodium soy sauce
- 2 tablespoons honey
- 2 cloves garlic, minced
- 1 tablespoon ginger, minced
- Sesame seeds for garnish

Instructions:

1. In a bowl, whisk together soy sauce, honey, garlic, and ginger.
2. Heat a large skillet over medium-high heat and stir-fry beef until browned.
3. Add broccoli and sauce, stir-fry for another 3-4 minutes.
4. Sprinkle with sesame seeds before serving.

Spaghetti Squash with Tomato Sauce

Ingredients:

- 1 spaghetti squash
- 2 cups low oxalate tomato sauce
- 1/2 cup grated Parmesan cheese
- Fresh basil leaves for garnish

Instructions:

1. Preheat your oven to 375°F (190°C).
2. Cut the squash in half lengthwise and scoop out the seeds.
3. Roast the squash halves, cut side down, for 35-45 minutes until tender.
4. Scrape the squash with a fork to create "spaghetti" strands.
5. Serve with heated tomato sauce and a sprinkle of Parmesan cheese and fresh basil.

Lemon Garlic Shrimp Scampi

Ingredients:

- 1 pound large shrimp, peeled and deveined
- 4 cloves garlic, minced
- Zest and juice of 1 lemon
- 2 tablespoons butter
- 2 tablespoons olive oil
- Fresh parsley for garnish

Instructions:

1. Heat butter and olive oil in a skillet over medium heat.
2. Add minced garlic and sauté until fragrant.
3. Add shrimp, lemon zest, and lemon juice. Cook until shrimp turn pink.
4. Garnish with fresh parsley before serving.

Stuffed Bell Peppers with Ground Turkey

Ingredients:

- 4 bell peppers, any color

- 1 pound ground turkey
- 1 cup cooked quinoa
- 1 cup low oxalate tomato sauce
- 1/2 cup diced onions
- 1/2 cup diced tomatoes
- 1/2 cup shredded mozzarella cheese
- Salt and pepper to taste

Instructions:

1. Preheat your oven to 350°F (175°C).
2. Cut the tops off the bell peppers and remove seeds.
3. In a skillet, cook ground turkey and onions until browned. Drain excess fat.
4. Mix in cooked quinoa, diced tomatoes, tomato sauce, salt, and pepper.
5. Stuff each bell pepper with the turkey mixture and top with mozzarella cheese.
6. Bake for 25-30 minutes until peppers are tender.

Portobello Mushroom Steaks

Ingredients:

- 4 large Portobello mushrooms

- 1/4 cup balsamic vinegar
- 2 tablespoons olive oil
- 2 cloves garlic, minced
- 1 teaspoon dried thyme
- Salt and pepper to taste

Instructions:

1. Clean mushrooms and remove stems.
2. In a bowl, whisk together balsamic vinegar, olive oil, garlic, thyme, salt, and pepper.
3. Brush the mixture onto both sides of the mushrooms.
4. Grill or broil the mushrooms for 5-7 minutes per side until tender.

Baked Cod with Herbed Crust

Ingredients:

- 4 cod fillets
- 1/2 cup breadcrumbs (from low oxalate bread)
- 2 tablespoons fresh parsley, chopped
- 2 tablespoons fresh dill, chopped
- 2 cloves garlic, minced
- 2 tablespoons olive oil

- Lemon wedges for garnish

Instructions:

1. Preheat your oven to 400°F (200°C).
2. In a bowl, mix breadcrumbs, parsley, dill, garlic, and olive oil.
3. Place cod fillets on a baking sheet and press the breadcrumb mixture on top.
4. Bake for 12-15 minutes until the fish flakes easily.
5. Serve with lemon wedges.

Zucchini Noodles with Pesto

Ingredients:

- 4 medium zucchinis, spiralized into noodles
- 1/2 cup pesto sauce
- Cherry tomatoes, halved, for garnish
- Grated Parmesan cheese for garnish

Instructions:

1. In a large skillet, sauté zucchini noodles until tender, about 3-4 minutes.
2. Toss with pesto sauce.

3. Garnish with cherry tomatoes and grated Parmesan cheese.

Quinoa-Stuffed Acorn Squash

Ingredients:

- 2 acorn squash, halved and seeds removed
- 1 cup quinoa, cooked
- 1/2 cup dried cranberries
- 1/4 cup chopped pecans
- 1 tablespoon maple syrup
- 1 teaspoon cinnamon
- Salt and pepper to taste

Instructions:

1. Preheat your oven to 375°F (190°C).
2. Place acorn squash halves on a baking sheet, cut side down, and roast for 30-35 minutes until tender.
3. In a bowl, combine cooked quinoa, dried cranberries, chopped pecans, maple syrup, cinnamon, salt, and pepper.
4. Stuff the roasted acorn squash halves with the quinoa mixture.

Thai Green Curry with Tofu

Ingredients:

- 1 package extra-firm tofu, cubed
- 1 can coconut milk
- 2 tablespoons green curry paste
- 1 red bell pepper, sliced
- 1 cup broccoli florets
- 1 tablespoon fish sauce (optional for flavor)
- Fresh basil leaves for garnish

Instructions:

1. In a large skillet, simmer coconut milk and green curry paste.
2. Add tofu, bell pepper, broccoli, and fish sauce (if using). Cook until vegetables are tender.
3. Serve hot, garnished with fresh basil leaves.

Roasted Cauliflower Steak

Ingredients:

- 1 large cauliflower head, sliced into "steaks"
- 2 tablespoons olive oil

- 1 teaspoon paprika
- 1/2 teaspoon cumin
- Salt and pepper to taste

Instructions:

1. Preheat your oven to 425°F (220°C).
2. Brush cauliflower steaks with olive oil and sprinkle with paprika, cumin, salt, and pepper.
3. Roast in the oven for 20-25 minutes until tender and slightly crispy.

Turkey Meatballs in Tomato Sauce

Ingredients:

- 1 pound ground turkey
- 1/2 cup breadcrumbs (from low oxalate bread)
- 1/4 cup grated Parmesan cheese
- 1 egg
- 2 cloves garlic, minced
- 1 can low oxalate tomato sauce
- Fresh basil for garnish

Instructions:

1. In a bowl, combine ground turkey, breadcrumbs, Parmesan cheese, egg, and minced garlic. Form into meatballs.
2. In a skillet, brown meatballs on all sides.
3. Add tomato sauce and simmer for 15-20 minutes until meatballs are cooked through.
4. Garnish with fresh basil before serving.

Sweet Potato and Black Bean Chili

Ingredients:

- 2 sweet potatoes, diced
- 1 can black beans, drained and rinsed
- 1 can low oxalate tomato sauce
- 1 tablespoon chili powder
- 1 teaspoon cumin
- Salt and pepper to taste

Instructions:

1. In a large pot, combine sweet potatoes, black beans, tomato sauce, chili powder, cumin, salt, and pepper.

2. Simmer for 20-25 minutes until sweet potatoes are tender.

Lemon Herb Tilapia

Ingredients:

- 4 tilapia fillets
- Zest and juice of 1 lemon
- 2 tablespoons olive oil
- Fresh thyme leaves
- Salt and pepper to taste

Instructions:

1. Preheat your oven to 375°F (190°C).
2. Place tilapia fillets on a baking sheet.
3. Mix lemon zest, lemon juice, olive oil, thyme leaves, salt, and pepper. Drizzle over the tilapia.
4. Bake for 15-20 minutes until fish flakes easily.

Ratatouille

Ingredients:

- 1 eggplant, diced

- 2 zucchinis, diced
- 1 red bell pepper, diced
- 1 yellow bell pepper, diced
- 1 onion, chopped
- 3 cloves garlic, minced
- 1 can low oxalate tomato sauce
- 1 teaspoon dried thyme
- 1 teaspoon dried oregano
- Salt and pepper to taste

Instructions:

1. In a large skillet, sauté onion and garlic until fragrant.
2. Add eggplant, zucchinis, red and yellow bell peppers, and cook until softened.
3. Stir in tomato sauce, thyme, oregano, salt, and pepper.
4. Simmer for 15-20 minutes until flavors meld together.

BBQ Pulled Chicken Lettuce Wraps

Ingredients:

- 2 chicken breasts

- 1 cup low oxalate BBQ sauce

- 1 head iceberg lettuce, leaves separated

- Coleslaw mix (optional for topping)

Instructions:

1. Place chicken breasts in a slow cooker and pour BBQ sauce over them.

2. Cook on low for 6-8 hours or until chicken is tender and can be easily shredded.

3. Serve the pulled chicken in lettuce leaves and top with coleslaw if desired.

Cabbage Roll Casserole

Ingredients:

- 1 pound ground beef

- 1 onion, chopped

- 1 cup cooked rice

- 1 can low oxalate tomato sauce

- 1 head cabbage, chopped

- 1 teaspoon paprika

- Salt and pepper to taste

Instructions:

1. In a skillet, brown ground beef and onion until cooked through.

2. Stir in cooked rice, tomato sauce, paprika, salt, and pepper.

3. Layer chopped cabbage in a baking dish and top with the meat mixture.

4. Bake at 350°F (175°C) for 30-35 minutes until cabbage is tender.

Chapter 5: Snacks and Appetizers

In Chapter 5, we're diving into a delectable array of snacks and appetizers designed to tantalize your taste buds without compromising your low oxalate diet. These bite-sized delights are perfect for gatherings or when you simply crave something savory or crunchy.

Guacamole with Veggie Sticks

Ingredients:

- 2 ripe avocados
- 1 ripe tomato, diced
- 1/2 red onion, finely chopped
- 1 clove garlic, minced
- Juice of 1 lime
- Salt and pepper to taste
- Assorted veggie sticks for dipping

Instructions:

1. Mash avocados in a bowl.
2. Add tomato, onion, garlic, and lime juice. Mix well.

3. Season with salt and pepper.

4. Serve with colorful veggie sticks for a healthy and creamy dip.

Roasted Red Pepper and Feta Dip

Ingredients:

- 2 red bell peppers
- 4 oz feta cheese, crumbled
- 2 cloves garlic, minced
- 2 tbsp olive oil
- Salt and pepper to taste
- Pita wedges or veggie slices for dipping

Instructions:

1. Roast red peppers until charred, then peel and chop.

2. Combine peppers, feta, garlic, and olive oil in a food processor.

3. Blend until smooth, season with salt and pepper.

4. Serve with pita or veggies for a flavorful dip.

Deviled Eggs

Ingredients:

- 6 hard-boiled eggs
- 2 tbsp mayonnaise
- 1 tsp Dijon mustard
- 1 tsp white vinegar
- Paprika and chives for garnish

Instructions:

1. Cut eggs in half lengthwise, remove yolks, and mash them.
2. Mix in mayonnaise, mustard, and vinegar.
3. Spoon mixture back into egg white halves.
4. Sprinkle with paprika and chives for extra flavor.

Cucumber Slices with Cream Cheese

Ingredients:

- 1 cucumber, sliced
- 4 oz cream cheese
- Fresh dill or chives for garnish

Instructions:

1. Spread cream cheese on cucumber slices.
2. Garnish with fresh dill or chives.
3. Enjoy these refreshing bites.

Kale Chips

Ingredients:

- Fresh kale leaves, stems removed
- Olive oil
- Salt and pepper

Instructions:

1. Preheat oven to 350°F (175°C).
2. Toss kale with olive oil, salt, and pepper.
3. Bake until crisp, about 10-15 minutes.
4. Let cool and savor the crispy goodness.

Edamame with Sea Salt

Ingredients:

- 2 cups edamame (frozen or fresh)
- Sea salt, to taste

Instructions:

1. Boil edamame in salted water until tender, about 5 minutes.
2. Drain and sprinkle with sea salt.
3. Pop them out of their pods for a healthy and satisfying snack.

Trail Mix with Low Oxalate Nuts

Ingredients:

- 1 cup almonds
- 1 cup cashews
- 1 cup dried cranberries
- 1/2 cup pumpkin seeds
- 1/2 cup sunflower seeds

Instructions:

1. Combine all ingredients in a bowl.
2. Mix well and portion into snack-sized bags for an energy-boosting trail mix.

Carrot and Hummus

Ingredients:

- Carrot sticks
- Hummus for dipping

Instructions:

1. Simply pair fresh carrot sticks with creamy hummus for a classic and nutritious combo.

Stuffed Mushrooms

Ingredients:

- Large mushrooms, cleaned and stems removed
- Cream cheese
- Chopped fresh herbs (e.g., parsley, thyme)
- Salt and pepper

Instructions:

1. Mix cream cheese, herbs, salt, and pepper.
2. Fill mushroom caps with the cream cheese mixture.
3. Bake until mushrooms are tender and tops are golden.

Greek Yogurt Dip with Veggies

Ingredients:

- 1 cup Greek yogurt
- 1 tsp lemon juice
- 1 clove garlic, minced
- Assorted fresh veggies for dipping

Instructions:

1. Combine yogurt, lemon juice, and garlic.
2. Serve as a healthy dip with fresh veggie sticks.

Baked Sweet Potato Fries

Ingredients:

- 2 sweet potatoes, cut into fries
- 2 tbsp olive oil
- Salt and paprika, to taste

Instructions:

1. Preheat oven to 425°F (220°C).
2. Toss sweet potato fries with olive oil, salt, and paprika.

3. Arrange on a baking sheet and bake until crispy, about 25-30 minutes.

Spinach and Artichoke Dip

Ingredients:

- 1 cup spinach, chopped and cooked
- 1 cup canned artichoke hearts, chopped
- 1 cup cream cheese
- 1/2 cup grated Parmesan cheese
- 1/2 cup sour cream
- 1 clove garlic, minced
- Salt and pepper, to taste

Instructions:

1. Mix spinach, artichoke hearts, cream cheese, Parmesan, sour cream, and garlic.
2. Season with salt and pepper.
3. Bake until bubbly and golden, then serve with crackers or veggies.

Almond and Coconut Energy Bites

Ingredients:

- 1 cup almonds
- 1/2 cup shredded coconut
- 1/4 cup honey
- 1/4 cup almond butter
- 1/2 tsp vanilla extract

Instructions:

1. Blend almonds and coconut in a food processor.
2. Add honey, almond butter, and vanilla. Blend until a sticky mixture forms.
3. Roll into bite-sized balls and chill.

Mini Caprese Skewers

Ingredients:

- Cherry tomatoes
- Fresh basil leaves
- Mozzarella balls
- Balsamic glaze for drizzling

Instructions:

1. Thread a tomato, basil leaf, and mozzarella ball onto skewers.

2. Drizzle with balsamic glaze for a flavorful appetizer.

Crispy Chickpeas

Ingredients:

*   1 can chickpeas, drained and rinsed
*   2 tbsp olive oil
*   Spices (e.g., paprika, cumin, garlic powder)
*   Salt and pepper, to taste

Instructions:

1. Toss chickpeas with olive oil, spices, salt, and pepper.

2. Bake at 400°F (200°C) until crunchy, about 30-40 minutes.

Avocado Deviled Eggs

Ingredients:

*   6 hard-boiled eggs

- 1 ripe avocado
- 2 tsp lime juice
- Paprika and cilantro for garnish

Instructions:

1. Cut eggs in half, remove yolks, and mash with avocado and lime juice.
2. Spoon mixture back into egg white halves.
3. Garnish with paprika and cilantro.

Smoked Salmon Roll-Ups

Ingredients:

- Smoked salmon slices
- Cream cheese
- Cucumber spears

Instructions:

1. Spread cream cheese on salmon slices.
2. Place a cucumber spear on each slice and roll up for an elegant appetizer.

Pita Chips with Roasted Red Pepper Hummus

Ingredients:

- Pita bread, cut into triangles
- Roasted red pepper hummus

Instructions:

1. Toast pita triangles until crisp.
2. Serve with flavorful roasted red pepper hummus.

Chapter 6: Desserts

In this chapter, we've curated delightful dessert recipes that are not only low in oxalates but also bursting with flavor. Whether you have a sweet tooth or want to impress your guests with these treats, you'll find something to satisfy your cravings.

Low Oxalate Chocolate Brownies

Ingredients:

- 1 cup almond flour
- 1/2 cup unsweetened cocoa powder
- 1/2 cup honey
- 1/4 cup coconut oil
- 2 eggs
- 1/2 teaspoon vanilla extract
- 1/4 teaspoon baking soda
- A pinch of salt

Instructions:

1. Preheat your oven to 350°F (175°C) and grease a baking dish.
2. In a mixing bowl, combine almond flour, cocoa powder, honey, coconut oil, eggs, vanilla extract, baking soda, and salt. Mix until well combined.
3. Pour the batter into the greased baking dish and spread it evenly.
4. Bake for 20-25 minutes or until a toothpick inserted in the center comes out mostly clean.
5. Allow the brownies to cool before cutting them into squares. Enjoy!

Berry Parfait

Ingredients:

- 1 cup low oxalate berries (e.g., blueberries, strawberries)
- 1 cup Greek yogurt
- 2 tablespoons honey
- 1/4 cup granola (ensure it's low oxalate)

Instructions:

1. In a glass or bowl, layer low oxalate berries, Greek yogurt, honey, and granola.
2. Repeat the layers as desired.
3. Top with a few extra berries and a drizzle of honey. Serve chilled.

Lemon Sorbet

Ingredients:

- 4 lemons, juiced and zested
- 1 cup water
- 1 cup honey

Instructions:

1. In a saucepan, combine water and honey. Heat over low heat until the honey dissolves. Allow it to cool.
2. Stir in lemon juice and zest.
3. Pour the mixture into an ice cream maker and churn according to the manufacturer's instructions.
4. Transfer the sorbet to an airtight container and freeze until firm. Scoop and enjoy!

Vanilla Chia Seed Pudding

Ingredients:

- 1/4 cup chia seeds
- 1 cup almond milk
- 1 teaspoon vanilla extract
- 2 tablespoons honey
- Fresh berries for topping

Instructions:

1. In a jar, mix chia seeds, almond milk, vanilla extract, and honey. Stir well.
2. Refrigerate for at least 2 hours or until the mixture thickens.
3. Serve in individual cups or bowls, topped with fresh berries.

Almond Flour Sugar Cookies

Ingredients:

- 2 cups almond flour
- 1/4 cup coconut oil
- 1/4 cup honey

- 1 egg
- 1/2 teaspoon vanilla extract
- 1/4 teaspoon baking soda
- A pinch of salt

Instructions:

1. Preheat your oven to 350°F (175°C) and line a baking sheet with parchment paper.
2. In a mixing bowl, combine almond flour, coconut oil, honey, egg, vanilla extract, baking soda, and salt. Mix until a dough forms.
3. Roll the dough into small balls and place them on the baking sheet.
4. Flatten each ball with the back of a fork.
5. Bake for 10-12 minutes or until the edges turn golden.
6. Allow the cookies to cool before serving.

Poached Pears in Red Wine

Ingredients:

- 4 ripe pears, peeled and cored
- 1 bottle of red wine (choose a low oxalate variety)

- 1 cup honey
- 2 cinnamon sticks
- 4 cloves
- Zest of 1 orange

Instructions:

1. In a large saucepan, combine red wine, honey, cinnamon sticks, cloves, and orange zest.
2. Bring the mixture to a simmer and add the pears.
3. Simmer gently for about 20-25 minutes, turning the pears occasionally until they are tender.
4. Remove the pears and let them cool.
5. Continue to simmer the wine mixture until it thickens into a syrup.
6. Serve the poached pears drizzled with the red wine syrup.

Chocolate Avocado Mousse

Ingredients:

- 2 ripe avocados
- 1/4 cup cocoa powder
- 1/4 cup honey

- 1 teaspoon vanilla extract
- A pinch of salt
- Fresh berries for garnish

Instructions:

1. In a blender or food processor, combine avocados, cocoa powder, honey, vanilla extract, and salt. Blend until smooth.
2. Divide the mousse into serving glasses and refrigerate for at least 30 minutes.
3. Garnish with fresh berries before serving.

Baked Apples with Cinnamon

Ingredients:

- 4 apples, cored
- 1/4 cup chopped low oxalate nuts (e.g., almonds or pecans)
- 2 tablespoons honey
- 1 teaspoon ground cinnamon
- 1/4 cup water

Instructions:

1. Preheat your oven to 350°F (175°C).
2. In a bowl, mix chopped nuts, honey, and ground cinnamon.
3. Stuff each cored apple with the nut mixture.
4. Place the apples in a baking dish, add water to the bottom of the dish, and cover with foil.
5. Bake for 30-40 minutes or until the apples are tender.
6. Serve warm.

Coconut Macaroons

Ingredients:

- 2 cups unsweetened shredded coconut
- 1/2 cup honey
- 2 egg whites
- 1 teaspoon vanilla extract
- A pinch of salt

Instructions:

1. Preheat your oven to 325°F (163°C) and line a baking sheet with parchment paper.

2. In a mixing bowl, combine shredded coconut, honey, egg whites, vanilla extract, and salt. Mix until well combined.

3. Drop spoonfuls of the mixture onto the prepared baking sheet.

4. Bake for 15-20 minutes or until the macaroons are lightly golden.

5. Allow them to cool before enjoying.

Strawberry Shortcake

Ingredients:

- 1 cup almond flour
- 1/4 cup coconut flour
- 1/4 cup honey
- 1/4 cup coconut oil
- 1/2 teaspoon baking soda
- A pinch of salt
- Fresh strawberries, sliced
- Coconut whipped cream (low oxalate) for topping

Instructions:

1. Preheat your oven to 350°F (175°C) and grease a cake pan.
2. In a mixing bowl, combine almond flour, coconut flour, honey, coconut oil, baking soda, and salt. Mix until it forms a dough.
3. Press the dough evenly into the cake pan and bake for 10-12 minutes or until lightly golden.
4. Allow the cake to cool, then slice it into squares.
5. Serve with fresh strawberries and a dollop of coconut whipped cream.

Pumpkin Pie Bites

Ingredients:

- 1 cup pumpkin puree
- 1/4 cup honey
- 1 teaspoon pumpkin pie spice
- 1/2 teaspoon vanilla extract
- A pinch of salt
- Low oxalate pie crust (store-bought or homemade)

Instructions:

1. Preheat your oven to 350°F (175°C).

2. In a bowl, combine pumpkin puree, honey, pumpkin pie spice, vanilla extract, and salt. Mix until smooth.

3. Roll out the pie crust and use a round cutter to make small circles.

4. Place each circle into a mini muffin tin and fill with the pumpkin mixture.

5. Bake for 15-20 minutes or until set.

6. Allow the pie bites to cool before serving.

Blueberry Almond Crisp

Ingredients:

- 2 cups low oxalate blueberries
- 1 cup almond flour
- 1/4 cup honey
- 1/4 cup coconut oil
- 1/4 cup sliced almonds
- 1/2 teaspoon cinnamon
- A pinch of salt

Instructions:

1. Preheat your oven to 350°F (175°C).

2. In a bowl, mix blueberries, honey, and a pinch of salt. Pour the mixture into a baking dish.

3. In another bowl, combine almond flour, coconut oil, sliced almonds, and cinnamon. Mix until crumbly.

4. Sprinkle the almond mixture over the blueberries.

5. Bake for 25-30 minutes or until the topping is golden and the berries are bubbling.

6. Let it cool slightly before serving.

Banana Ice Cream

Ingredients:

- 4 ripe bananas, sliced and frozen
- 1/4 cup almond milk
- 1 teaspoon vanilla extract

Instructions:

1. Place frozen banana slices in a blender or food processor.

2. Add almond milk and vanilla extract.

3. Blend until you achieve a creamy ice cream consistency.

4. Serve immediately as a guilt-free frozen treat.

Lemon Poppy Seed Cake

Ingredients:

- 2 cups almond flour
- 1/4 cup coconut flour
- 1/4 cup honey
- 1/4 cup coconut oil
- 2 eggs
- Zest and juice of 2 lemons
- 1 teaspoon baking soda
- 1 tablespoon poppy seeds
- A pinch of salt

Instructions:

1. Preheat your oven to 350°F (175°C) and grease a cake pan.

2. In a mixing bowl, combine almond flour, coconut flour, honey, coconut oil, eggs, lemon zest, lemon

juice, baking soda, poppy seeds, and salt. Mix until well combined.

3. Pour the batter into the greased cake pan.

4. Bake for 25-30 minutes or until a toothpick inserted in the center comes out clean.

5. Allow the cake to cool before slicing and serving.

Rice Pudding with Berries

Ingredients:

- 1 cup cooked white rice (low oxalate)
- 1 cup almond milk
- 1/4 cup honey
- 1 teaspoon vanilla extract
- 1/2 teaspoon ground cinnamon
- Mixed berries for topping

Instructions:

1. In a saucepan, combine cooked rice, almond milk, honey, vanilla extract, and ground cinnamon.

2. Cook over low heat, stirring occasionally, until the mixture thickens.

3. Remove from heat and let it cool.

4. Serve with a generous topping of mixed berries.

Dark Chocolate Bark with Nuts

Ingredients:

- 1 cup low oxalate dark chocolate chips
- 1/4 cup chopped low oxalate nuts (e.g., almonds or walnuts)
- A pinch of sea salt

Instructions:

1. Line a baking sheet with parchment paper.
2. Melt the dark chocolate chips in a microwave or using a double boiler.
3. Pour the melted chocolate onto the parchment paper and spread it into a thin layer.
4. Sprinkle chopped nuts and a pinch of sea salt over the chocolate.
5. Allow it to cool and harden in the refrigerator for about an hour.
6. Break into pieces and enjoy your homemade chocolate bark.

Mango Sorbet

Ingredients:

- 2 ripe mangoes, peeled and diced
- 1/4 cup honey
- Juice of 1 lime
- 1/4 cup water

Instructions:

1. In a blender, combine diced mangoes, honey, lime juice, and water.
2. Blend until smooth.
3. Transfer the mixture to an ice cream maker and churn according to the manufacturer's instructions.
4. Freeze until firm and scoop to serve.

Pecan Pie Bites

Ingredients:

- 1 cup pecans, chopped
- 1/4 cup honey
- 2 eggs
- 2 tablespoons coconut oil

- 1 teaspoon vanilla extract
- A pinch of salt
- Low oxalate pie crust (store-bought or homemade)

Instructions:

1. Preheat your oven to 350°F (175°C) and grease a mini muffin tin.
2. In a bowl, mix chopped pecans, honey, eggs, coconut oil, vanilla extract, and a pinch of salt.
3. Roll out the pie crust and use a round cutter to make small circles.
4. Press each circle into the mini muffin tin.
5. Fill each crust with the pecan mixture.
6. Bake for 12-15 minutes or until set.
7. Allow the pecan pie bites to cool before serving.

CONCLUSION

Throughout this journey, you've discovered an extensive collection of recipes spanning breakfast, lunch, dinner, snacks, and desserts. Each dish was carefully crafted to minimize oxalate content while maximizing flavor and nutrition. From the comforting aroma of a steaming bowl of cauliflower soup to the zesty burst of flavor in a Mediterranean-inspired salad, these recipes have showcased the culinary artistry that can be achieved within the constraints of a low oxalate diet.

But this book is more than just recipes. It's a guide that empowers you to make informed choices about your dietary habits, leading to improved well-being and overall health. It's a testament to the idea that healthy eating can be an enjoyable and fulfilling experience.

As you turn the final page, remember that your low oxalate journey is far from over. It's a lifestyle, a commitment to your health and vitality. You now possess the knowledge and skills to continue exploring and creating low oxalate dishes that resonate with your palate. Keep experimenting, keep savoring, and keep prioritizing your well-being.

In closing, I want to express my gratitude for joining us on this culinary adventure. I hope this recipe book has not only filled your plates but also enriched your life. May your low oxalate journey be a path to health, happiness, and delicious discoveries.

Wishing you all the best on your ongoing culinary adventures.